STAGE 3 KIDNEY DISEASE DIET COOKBOOK FOR OLDER

MEN AND WOMEN

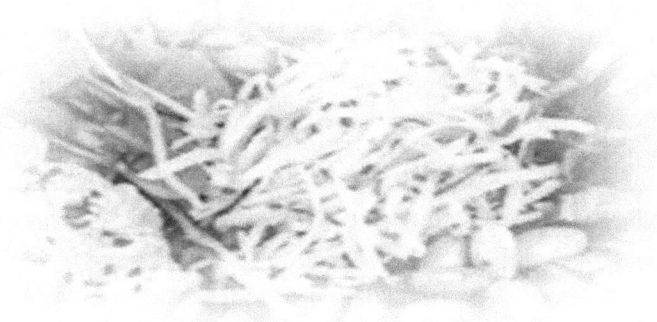

Healthy and Delicious Low Sodium, Low Phosphorus and Low Potassium Recipes to Manage Chronic Kidney Disease

David T. Salcedo

Copyright © 2023 by David T. Salcedo

Table of Contents

INTRODUCTION

Sarah, a vivacious older woman, found herself battling with a health problem she had not anticipated. A regular checkup revealed that she had Stage 3 kidney disease, putting her in a state of uncertainty. When she learned of her diagnosis, Sarah resolved not to let it define her; instead, she set out on a journey to reclaim her health.

Sarah dug into studying the complicated dance of kidneys in sustaining overall health, armed with resolve. She read medical journals, spoke with dietitians, and soaked in information like a sponge. She understood that her diet could play a critical part in managing the progression of her disease after learning about the effects of sodium, potassium, phosphorus, and protein on kidney function.

Sarah's kitchen underwent a makeover. High-sodium condiments and processed foods were eliminated and replaced with kidney-friendly alternatives. She experimented with a variety of fresh vegetables and fruits, discovering their distinct flavors and nutritional benefits. Sarah also experimented with culinary methods, perfecting the skill of grilling, steaming, and roasting to retain nutrients without sacrificing flavor.

Sarah set out on a culinary expedition, armed with newfound knowledge and a revitalized kitchen. She developed meals that not only complied with her dietary constraints but were also flavorful. Each meal became a celebration of sustenance and wellbeing, from vivid smoothie bowls for breakfast to flavorful salads for lunch and nourishing, protein-rich meals.

Changing to a kidney-friendly diet presented hurdles, which Sarah confronted full on. Dining out with friends became an opportunity to educate others about her dietary requirements, and she uncovered hidden treasures on menus that matched her health goals. Sarah's fortitude shone through, turning each setback into an opportunity for growth.

Sarah was not alone on this journey. She told her story to friends, relatives, and an online community. Her tale resonated with others on similar health journeys, forming a network of encouragement and support. Sarah became an inspiration, demonstrating that with perseverance and the appropriate attitude, it is possible to manage and even thrive with Stage 3 Kidney Disease.

Sarah's dedication to a kidney-friendly lifestyle brought astounding effects over time. Her energy levels increased, and routine examinations revealed that her renal function was stable. Sarah's tale was not only about dealing with a health condition, but also about the transformative potential of adopting a nutritious lifestyle.

Sarah is no longer a victim of her condition, but rather a triumphant navigator of her health path. Her kitchen, which was previously a source of anxiety, is now a hive of creativity and life. Sarah reinvented her health story through dietary changes and tenacity, demonstrating that a diagnosis does not determine one's fate. She continues to savor the richness of life with each wholesome meal, greeting each day with appreciation and increased vitality.

Kidney Function Overview

The kidneys, a pair of bean-shaped organs positioned just below the rib cage on either side of the spine, play an important function in the overall health of the body. These extraordinary organs are in charge of a plethora of functions that contribute to the body's homeostasis, filtration, and waste disposal. An overview of kidney function entails a complex interaction of physiological processes that ensure the body's internal milieu remains steady.

1. Blood Filtration

One of the kidneys' principal duties is to continuously filter the blood. These organs process 120 to 150 quarts of blood per day, removing 1 to 2 quarts of waste and extra fluid. This waste, combined with toxins, excess salts, and urea, is what we call urine.

2. Electrolyte Regulation

The kidneys play an important role in regulating the body's electrolyte balance, which includes salt, potassium, and phosphate. These electrolytes are necessary for a variety of physiological activities, including nerve impulse transmission, muscular contraction, and acid-base homeostasis. The kidneys fine-tune the concentration of these electrolytes in the blood through selective reabsorption and excretion.

3. Blood Pressure Control

Kidneys play a critical function in blood pressure regulation. Specialized cells in the kidneys monitor blood pressure and release the enzyme renin in response. Renin works as a catalyst in the conversion of angiotensinogen to angiotensin I, which results in the creation of angiotensin II, a strong vasoconstrictor. This system regulates blood pressure by altering blood vessel diameter.

4. Erythropoiesis Control

The kidneys create erythropoietin, a hormone that encourages the bone marrow to make red blood cells. In reaction to low oxygen levels in the blood, erythropoietin is released, guaranteeing an adequate supply of red blood cells to transport oxygen throughout the body.

5. Balance of Acids and Bases

The pH equilibrium of biological fluids must be maintained for optimal physiological function. The kidneys maintain acid-base equilibrium by excreting hydrogen ions selectively and reabsorbing bicarbonate ions. This procedure keeps the blood from becoming overly acidic or alkaline.

6. Detoxification and Waste Removal

By filtering metabolic waste products, medicines, and other chemicals from the blood, the kidneys act as the body's natural detoxification system. These waste products are then expelled as urine, keeping hazardous compounds from accumulating in the body.

7. Glucose Control

While the kidneys' primary function is not glucose management, they do help to maintain blood glucose homeostasis by reabsorbing glucose during the filtration process. In hyperglycemia, such as diabetes, the kidneys may be unable to reabsorb all of the glucose, resulting in its presence in the urine.

What is Stage 3 kidney disease?

Stage 3 kidney disease, also known as mild chronic kidney disease (CKD), is a stage in the decrease of kidney function. The glomerular filtration rate (GFR), which measures how successfully the kidneys filter waste from the blood, is often used to determine the stages of CKD. renal function is substantially impaired in Stage 3, but the condition has not advanced to severe or end-stage renal disease.

Key Features of Stage 3 kidney disease
1.GFR Variables

- Stage 3a: GFR is 45-59 mL/min/1.73 m2.

- Stage 3b: GFR ranges from 30-44 mL/min/1.73 m2.

2.Symptoms range from mild to moderate.

- People with Stage 3 renal disease may or may not have symptoms.

- Some of the most common symptoms are weariness, changes in urine output, swelling (edema), and minor back pain.

3. Risk Factors Increased

- People with Stage 3 CKD are more likely to have consequences such as anemia, bone disease, and cardiovascular problems.

4. Management and Lifestyle Changes

- A focus on underlying disorders that contribute to kidney disease, including hypertension and diabetes.

- Implementation of dietary adjustments to reduce salt, phosphorus, and potassium intake.

- Keeping track of and controlling other risk factors including high blood pressure and diabetes.

5. Medical supervision

- Blood tests (serum creatinine and estimated GFR) and urine tests are used to assess renal function on a regular basis.

- Controlling risk factors to slow the progression of renal disease.

Causes of Stage 3 Kidney Disease

1.Chronic Illnesses

- Hypertension (High Blood Pressure): High blood pressure for an extended period of time can damage the blood vessels in the kidneys, limiting their ability to function effectively.

- Diabetes: Uncontrolled diabetes can cause diabetic nephropathy, or damage to the tiny blood vessels in the kidneys.

2.Primary Kidney Diseases

- Glomerulonephritis: Glomeruli, the kidney's filtering units, can become inflamed, causing kidney damage.

- Polycystic Kidney Disease: An inherited condition in which fluid-filled cysts grow in the kidneys, interfering with their function over time.

3. Obstruction of the Urinary Tract

- Enlarged Prostate: An enlarged prostate in men can cause urinary blockage, resulting in kidney damage.

- Kidney Stones: Recurrent kidney stones can clog the urinary tract and impair kidney function.

4.Other Factors

- Autoimmune Diseases: Lupus and certain infections can both cause kidney damage.

- Long-Term Use of Certain Medications: Long-term use of nonsteroidal anti-inflammatory medications (NSAIDs) and some antibiotics can contribute to kidney impairment.

Symptoms of Stage 3 kidney disease

1.Fatigue and weakness are caused by anemia, which is caused by a decrease in erythropoietin production.

2.Fluid retention, typically seen in the hands, ankles, and around the eyes, causes swelling (edema).

3.Urination Changes

- An increase in frequency, particularly at night.

- Protein loss is indicated by foamy or frothy urine.

- Urine that is darker or contains blood.

4.Hypertension (High Blood Pressure): High blood pressure can both cause and exacerbate kidney disease.

5.Back Pain: Although not always present, discomfort or pain around the kidneys.

Preventive Measures for Stage 3 kidney disease

1.Manage the Subsequent Conditions

- Blood Pressure Control: Hypertension should be monitored and managed on a regular basis.

- Diabetes management includes regular blood sugar monitoring and adherence to treatment recommendations.

- Weight Control: Maintain a healthy weight to lower your risk of diabetes and hypertension.

2.Choices for a Healthy Lifestyle

- Healthy Diet: Eat a kidney-friendly diet reduced in salt, phosphorus, and potassium.

- Regular Physical Activity: Engage in regular physical activity to support general health and weight management.

- Avoid Smoking and Drink Moderately: Both smoking and excessive alcohol use can cause kidney impairment.

3.Regular Medical Exams

- Regular Kidney Function Tests: Blood and urine tests are used to assess kidney function on a regular basis.

- Medication Review: Discuss medications with your healthcare professional on a regular basis to avoid potentially kidney-damaging drugs.

4.Hydration

- Adequate Fluid Intake: Stay hydrated to help prevent kidney stones and promote overall kidney function.

5.Treatment of Infections as Soon as Possible

- Prompt Treatment: Treat infections as soon as possible to prevent them from spreading to the kidneys.

6.Genetic Guidance

- Polycystic Kidney Disease: If a family history exists, genetic counseling and routine testing should be considered.

Understanding The Progression And Impact Of Stage 3 Kidney Disease

Chronic kidney disease (CKD) is a degenerative disorder that progresses in stages, with Stage 3 being a watershed moment when the impact on kidney function becomes more severe. Understanding the evolution and impact of Stage 3 kidney disease is critical for both individuals and healthcare professionals, as it guides management techniques and decisions to reduce its impacts.

1. Stage 3 Kidney Disease Progression

Gradual Loss of Kidney Function

- The glomerular filtration rate (GFR), which assesses the kidneys' ability to filter waste from the blood, decreases moderately in Stage 3.

- This stage, which is divided into Stage 3a (GFR 45-59 mL/min/1.73 m2) and Stage 3b (GFR 30-44 mL/min/1.73 m2), denotes a severe decline in the kidneys' filtering ability.

Increasing Complications and Risks

- The risk of problems increases as Stage 3 continues. People may notice weariness, changes in urine output, swelling (edema), and slight back pain.

- The increased vulnerability to anemia, bone disease, and cardiovascular difficulties highlights the importance of close monitoring.

Contributing Factors' Influence

- Common factors of CKD, such as hypertension and diabetes, continue to play an important role in disease progression.

- Lifestyle variables, such as food and exercise, are becoming increasingly important in controlling chronic disorders in order to decrease the course of renal disease.

2. Impact on Life Quality

Physical Signs and Symptoms

- As kidney function diminishes, fatigue and weakness may become more noticeable, affecting an individual's daily activities and overall energy levels.

- Edema (swelling) of the extremities may occur, and alterations in urine output may interfere with normal body processes.

Emotional and Mental Health

- The chronic nature of renal disease, as well as its potential impact on daily living, can lead to emotional discomfort and mental health issues.

- Coping with the uncertainty of a progressing condition can lead to worry or despair, emphasizing the significance of holistic care that treats both physical and emotional components.

Lifestyle Changes

- In Stage 3, dietary limitations and adjustments become increasingly important. Controlling salt, potassium, and phosphorus consumption is critical for preventing complications and slowing disease development.

- Regular medication monitoring and adjustments become normal, necessitating a commitment to self-care and adherence to prescribed therapies.

3. Medical Management and Future Prospects

Multidisciplinary Strategy

- Management of Stage 3 kidney disease requires a team effort from healthcare specialists such as nephrologists, nutritionists, and primary care clinicians.

- Regular medical monitoring, including blood tests, urine tests, and imaging investigations, aids in tracking kidney function and assessing the effectiveness of therapies.

Reducing Progression and Avoiding Complications

- Managing risk factors including hypertension and diabetes becomes critical in reducing the progression of renal disease.

- Early intervention, lifestyle changes, and medication adherence are all important factors in avoiding problems and improving overall outcomes.

Advanced Care Consideration

- Discussions concerning potential future interventions, such as renal replacement therapy (dialysis or kidney transplantation), may arise in later stages of Stage 3 CKD. These conversations are critical for making informed decisions and ensuring that individuals are actively participating in their care planning.

The Importance of Diet in Kidney Health Management

Maintaining optimal kidney health is inextricably linked to lifestyle decisions, with nutrition being one of the most crucial. Dietary habits are important in controlling kidney health for more than just nutrition; they have an important role in reducing the progression of renal disease, preventing complications, and improving general well-being. This holistic approach to kidney health entails learning about the effects of numerous nutrients on the kidneys and following a kidney-friendly diet.

1. Nutrient Intake Balance

Sodium Management

- Excess salt consumption can lead to fluid retention and high blood pressure, both of which are harmful to kidney health. Kidney-friendly diets prioritize sodium reduction, which is generally accomplished by avoiding processed foods and opting for fresh, whole foods.

Controlling Potassium Levels

- Impaired kidney function may cause a buildup of potassium in the blood, increasing the risk of heart-related problems. Maintaining electrolyte balance requires controlling potassium intake by limiting high-potassium meals.

Understanding Phosphorus

- Elevated phosphorus levels in those with renal disease can cause bone and cardiovascular problems. Phosphorus management entails eating foods with decreased phosphorus content and maybe utilizing phosphate binders as suggested by healthcare specialists.

Protein Balance

- While protein is necessary for good health, too much protein can strain the kidneys. The emphasis in kidney disease management is frequently on maintaining a moderate protein intake to lessen the stress on the kidneys.

2. Management of Fluids

Proper Hydration

- Adequate fluid intake is critical for kidney function since it aids in the elimination of waste materials from the body. Individuals with kidney illness, on the other hand, may need to limit their fluid consumption based on their specific condition and the advise of healthcare professionals.

Fluid Retention Monitoring

- Kidney-friendly diets stress the importance of monitoring and managing fluid retention. Individuals can maintain an optimum fluid balance by limiting sodium consumption and paying attention to thirst cues.

3. Kidney-Friendly Recipes

Fruits and vegetables

- Consuming a variety of fruits and vegetables gives important vitamins, minerals, and antioxidants. Choices should, however, be customized to specific dietary constraints, notably in terms of potassium content.

Low-Phosphorus Foods and Whole Grains

- Choosing whole grains and low-phosphorus foods promotes a balanced diet while meeting the unique needs of those with kidney disease.

Sources of Lean Protein

- Choosing lean protein sources, such as poultry, fish, and plant-based proteins, aids in protein management while also delivering vital amino acids for overall health.

4. Diet Plans for Individuals

Dietitian Consultation

- Developing a tailored nutrition plan is critical for maintaining kidney health. Renal nutritionists can provide individualized advice based on an individual's specific needs, considering parameters such as GFR, medications, and comorbid diseases.

Monitoring and Modification

- Regular monitoring of kidney function via blood and urine testing allows healthcare providers to evaluate the efficacy of dietary changes. Dietary adjustments can then be made as needed.

5. Avoiding Complications and Improving Well-Being:

Kidney Disease Progression Slowing

- When paired with other lifestyle changes, a kidney-friendly diet can help to halt the course of renal disease. This is especially important in the early phases, when treatments might have a big impact.

Complication Risk Reduction

- Dietary choices can help lower the risk of problems linked with renal disease, such as cardiovascular disease, bone disease, and anemia.

Improving Overall Life Quality

- A well-managed diet not only promotes kidney health but also improves overall quality of life. Individuals can feel more empowered in managing their disease and preserving a sense of well-being by addressing nutritional elements.

6. Educational Resources and Assistance

Individual Empowerment

- Providing kidney disease patients and caregivers with educational resources on kidney-friendly diets enables them to make educated decisions and actively engage in their care.

Community Support

Participating in supportive networks and receiving professional advice develops a collaborative approach to controlling kidney health through food. Shared experiences and knowledge help to provide a more complete understanding of nutritional control.

Understanding the Role of Key Nutrients in Kidney Health

Maintaining kidney health necessitates a careful balance of critical nutrients that promote optimal function and aid in the management of disorders such as chronic kidney disease (CKD). The major nutrients listed below play critical roles in promoting kidney health, and understanding their properties is critical for developing a kidney-friendly diet.

1. Sodium

- Function: Sodium, a component of salt, is essential for fluid balance and blood pressure regulation.

Characteristics include

- A high salt intake can cause fluid retention, which increases the stress on the kidneys.

- Kidney-friendly diets frequently decrease sodium intake to assist manage blood pressure and fluid retention.

- High salt content is typical in processed foods, canned items, and restaurant-prepared meals.

2. Potassium

- Function: Potassium is required for neuron and muscle cell function, including heart function.

Characteristics include

- High potassium levels can be harmful to the heart and other organs in people who have compromised renal function.

- Kidney-friendly diets frequently include monitoring and managing potassium consumption through the selection of low-potassium foods.

- Potassium is found naturally in fruits, vegetables, and certain legumes.

3. Phosphorus

- Function: Phosphorus is essential for bone health, energy metabolism, and pH equilibrium.

Characteristics include

- In kidney disease, inadequate phosphorus excretion can result in increased blood levels, contributing to bone and cardiovascular problems.

- Kidney-friendly diets emphasize low-phosphorus foods and may include the use of phosphate binders.

- Phosphorus-rich additives are commonly found in processed and packaged foods.

4. Protein

- Function: Proteins are important for overall health, tissue repair, and immunological function.

Characteristics include

- While protein is necessary, excessive protein consumption can strain the kidneys, especially in people with renal disease.

- Kidney-friendly diets frequently include limiting protein intake to lessen the stress on the kidneys.

- Lean protein sources such as poultry, fish, and plant-based choices are prioritized.

5. Fluids

- Function: Adequate fluid intake is necessary for kidney function, since it aids in the elimination of waste materials from the body.

Characteristics include

- People with kidney illness may need to limit their fluid consumption based on their unique condition and the advice of their healthcare professional.

- It is critical to monitor fluid retention and alter intake accordingly in order to maintain proper fluid balance.

- Caffeine and alcohol can cause dehydration and should be avoided in some circumstances.

6. Calcium

- Function: Calcium is essential for bone health, blood coagulation, and neuron communication.

Characteristics include

- • Kidney disease can affect bone health by disrupting calcium and phosphorus balance.

- Kidney-friendly diets strive for an appropriate calcium-to-phosphorus ratio, which is commonly achieved by dietary changes or supplementation.

- Calcium is commonly found in dairy products, leafy greens, and fortified foods.

7. D vitamin

- Function: Vitamin D is required for calcium absorption and bone health.

Characteristics include

- People with kidney disease may have impaired vitamin D activation, which could lead to bone problems.

- Kidney-friendly diets may include vitamin D supplementation as well as monitoring.

- Vitamin D intake is increased by sun exposure and dietary sources such as fatty fish and fortified meals.

Foods to Avoid or Limit on a Kidney Disease Stage 3 Diet

Food to Eat

1. Low-Potassium Fruit

   - Apples

   - Berries (strawberries, blueberries)

   - Pineapple

   - Cranberries

2. Low-Phosphorus Vegetables

   - Cauliflower

   - Cabbage

   - Bell peppers

   - Kale

3. Lean Protein Sources

   - Skinless poultry

   - Fish (especially those lower in phosphorus, like salmon)

   - Eggs

   - Plant-based proteins (tofu, legumes)

4. Whole Grains

   - Quinoa

   - Brown rice

- Oats

- Whole wheat products in moderation

5. Low-Fat Dairy or Dairy Alternatives

- Low-fat or fat-free milk

- Greek yogurt

- Almond milk (unsweetened)

6. Healthy Fats

- Olive oil

- Avocado

- Nuts and seeds in moderation

7. Herbs and Spices

- Use herbs and spices to add flavor without added sodium.

8. Limited Fluids

- Follow individualized fluid restrictions as advised by healthcare professionals.

Foods to Limit or Avoid

1. High-Potassium Fruits

   - Bananas

   - Oranges

   - Potatoes

   - Tomatoes and tomato-based products

2. High-Phosphorus Foods

   - Dairy products high in phosphorus (cheese, yogurt)

   - Nuts and seeds

   - Processed foods with phosphorus additives

3. Red and Processed Meats

   - Beef

   - Pork

   - Processed meats (sausages, bacon)

4. High-Sodium Foods

   - Processed foods

   - Canned soups and broths

   - Pickled and cured foods

5. Whole Grains in Excess

- Limit whole grains if phosphorus levels are a concern.

6. Excessive Protein

- Moderation is key; avoid excessive intake of protein-rich foods.

7. High-Potassium and Phosphorus Beverages

- Colas

- Certain fruit juices (orange, tomato)

- Energy drinks

8. Alcohol

- Limit alcohol intake, as it can impact kidney function.

CHAPTER 1

Breakfast Recipes

1. Quinoa Breakfast Bowl

Ingredients

- 1/2 cup quinoa (rinsed)

- 1 cup water

- 1/4 cup blueberries

- 1/4 cup sliced strawberries

- 1 tablespoon chopped almonds

- 1 teaspoon honey

Preparation

1. Cook quinoa in water according to package instructions.

2. Top cooked quinoa with blueberries, strawberries, almonds, and drizzle with honey.

Nutritional Information

- Calories: 300

- Protein: 10g

- Fiber: 5g

- Potassium: 180mg

- Phosphorus: 150mg

Serving Size: 1 bowl

Preparation Time: 15 minutes

2. Egg White Veggie Omelette

Ingredients

- 3 egg whites

- 1/4 cup diced bell peppers

- 1/4 cup diced tomatoes

- 1 tablespoon chopped spinach

- 1 teaspoon olive oil

Preparation

1. Whisk egg whites in a bowl.

2. Sauté vegetables in olive oil until tender.

3. Pour egg whites over vegetables and cook until set.

Nutritional Information

- Calories: 120

- Protein: 15g

- Fiber: 2g

- Potassium: 250mg

- Phosphorus: 100mg

Serving Size: 1 omelette

Preparation Time: 10 minutes

3. Buckwheat Pancakes with Berries

Ingredients

- 1/2 cup buckwheat flour

- 1/2 cup almond milk

- 1 egg

- 1/2 teaspoon baking powder

- 1/4 cup blueberries

- 1/4 cup raspberries

Preparation

1. Mix buckwheat flour, almond milk, egg, and baking powder.

2. Cook pancakes on a griddle.

3. Top with fresh berries.

Nutritional Information

- Calories: 250

- Protein: 8g

- Fiber: 5g

- Potassium: 180mg

- Phosphorus: 120mg

Serving Size: 2 pancakes

Preparation Time: 20 minutes

4. Greek Yogurt Parfait

Ingredients

- 1/2 cup low-fat Greek yogurt

- 1/4 cup granola (low-phosphorus)

- 1/4 cup sliced peaches

- 1 tablespoon chopped walnuts

Preparation

1. Layer Greek yogurt with granola, peaches, and walnuts.

Nutritional Information

- Calories: 200

- Protein: 12g

- Fiber: 3g

- Potassium: 150mg

- Phosphorus: 100mg

Serving Size: 1 parfait

Preparation Time: 5 minutes

5. Sweet Potato Hash with Poached Eggs

Ingredients

- 1/2 cup diced sweet potatoes

- 1/4 cup diced red onions

- 1/4 cup chopped bell peppers

- 2 poached eggs

Preparation

1. Sauté sweet potatoes, red onions, and bell peppers until tender.

2. Top with poached eggs.

Nutritional Information

- Calories: 220
- Protein: 12g
- Fiber: 4g
- Potassium: 280mg
- Phosphorus: 130mg

Serving Size: 1 serving

Preparation Time: 15 minutes

6. Chia Seed Pudding with Almond Milk

Ingredients

- 2 tablespoons chia seeds

- 1/2 cup unsweetened almond milk

- 1/4 teaspoon vanilla extract

- 1/4 cup diced mango

- 1 tablespoon shredded coconut

Preparation

1. Mix chia seeds, almond milk, and vanilla extract.

2. Leave it to stay for few hours or overnight until it thickens.

3. Top with diced mango and shredded coconut.

Nutritional Information

- Calories: 180

- Protein: 5g

- Fiber: 10g

- Potassium: 150mg

- Phosphorus: 80mg

Serving Size: 1 serving

Preparation Time: 5 minutes (plus soaking time)

7. Turkey and Vegetable Breakfast Wrap

Ingredients

- 1 whole-grain tortilla

- 2 ounces turkey breast (low-sodium)

- 1/4 cup sautéed spinach and tomatoes

- 1 tablespoon hummus

Preparation

1. Layer turkey, sautéed vegetables, and hummus on a tortilla.

2. Roll into a wrap.

Nutritional Information

- Calories: 250

- Protein: 18g

- Fiber: 5g

- Potassium: 200mg

- Phosphorus: 150mg

Serving Size: 1 wrap

Preparation Time: 10 minutes

8. Cottage Cheese and Fruit Bowl

Ingredients

- 1/2 cup low-fat cottage cheese

- 1/4 cup diced pineapple

- 1/4 cup sliced strawberries

- 1 tablespoon sunflower seeds

Preparation

1. Combine cottage cheese, pineapple, strawberries, and sunflower seeds.

Nutritional Information

- Calories: 200

- Protein: 15g

- Fiber: 2g

- Potassium: 220mg

- Phosphorus: 120mg

Serving Size: 1 bowl

Preparation Time: 5 minutes

9. Oatmeal with Cinnamon and Apple Slices

Ingredients

- 1/2 cup old-fashioned oats

- 1 cup water or low-phosphorus milk

- 1/2 teaspoon cinnamon

- 1/2 apple, sliced

Preparation

1. Cook oats with water or milk and cinnamon.

2. Top with sliced apple.

Nutritional Information

- Calories: 220

- Protein: 7g

- Fiber: 5g

- Potassium: 150mg

- Phosphorus: 100mg

Serving Size: 1 serving

Preparation Time: 10 minutes

10. Smoothie Bowl with Spinach and Berries

Ingredients

- 1/2 cup spinach leaves

- 1/2 cup mixed berries (blueberries, raspberries)

- 1/2 banana

- 1/2 cup unsweetened almond milk

- 1 tablespoon chia seeds

Preparation

1. Blend spinach, berries, banana, and almond milk until smooth.

2. It should be poured into a bowl and topped with chia seeds.

Nutritional Information

- Calories: 180

- Protein: 5g

- Fiber: 8g

- Potassium: 250mg

- Phosphorus: 80mg

Serving Size: 1 bowl

Preparation Time: 5 minutes

CHAPTER 2

Lunch Recipes

1. Grilled Chicken and Vegetable Skewers

Ingredients

- 4 ounces grilled chicken breast

- Bell peppers, cherry tomatoes, and zucchini chunks

- 1 tablespoon olive oil

- Rosemary, thyme and garlic powder should be example of herbs and spices to use.

Preparation

1. Thread chicken and vegetables onto skewers.

2. Brush with olive oil and sprinkle with herbs.

3. Grill until chicken is cooked through.

Nutritional Information

- Calories: 250

- Protein: 30g

- Fiber: 4g

- Potassium: 300mg

- Phosphorus: 200mg

Serving Size: 1 serving

Preparation Time: 20 minutes

2. Salmon and Quinoa Salad

Ingredients

- 4 ounces baked or grilled salmon

- 1/2 cup cooked quinoa

- Mixed greens

- Cherry tomatoes, cucumber slices

- lemon juice and olive oil should be used as lemon vinaigrette dressing.

Preparation

1. Flake salmon and place on a bed of mixed greens.

2. Add cooked quinoa, cherry tomatoes, and cucumber.

3. Drizzle with lemon vinaigrette.

Nutritional Information

- Calories: 300

- Protein: 25g

- Fiber: 5g

- Potassium: 400mg

- Phosphorus: 220mg

Serving Size: 1 salad

Preparation Time: 25 minutes

3. Vegetarian Stir-Fry with Tofu

Ingredients

- 1 cup firm tofu, cubed

- Assorted stir-fry vegetables (broccoli, bell peppers, snap peas)

- Low-sodium soy sauce

- 1 tablespoon sesame oil

- Brown rice (1/2 cup cooked)

Preparation

1. Sauté tofu until golden.

2. Add vegetables and stir-fry until tender.

3. It should be Drizzled with soy sauce and sesame oil.

4. Serve over brown rice.

Nutritional Information

- Calories: 280

- Protein: 20g

- Fiber: 6g

- Potassium: 350mg

- Phosphorus: 180mg

Serving Size: 1 serving

Preparation Time: 30 minutes

4. Mediterranean Chicken Wrap

Ingredients

- 4 ounces grilled chicken strips

- Whole-grain wrap

- Hummus

- Cherry tomatoes, cucumber slices, feta cheese

- Kalamata olives

Preparation

1. Spread hummus on the wrap.

2. Add grilled chicken, vegetables, feta, and olives.

3. Roll into a wrap.

Nutritional Information

- Calories: 320

- Protein: 25g

- Fiber: 6g

- Potassium: 250mg

- Phosphorus: 200mg

Serving Size: 1 wrap

Preparation Time: 15 minutes

5. Lentil and Vegetable Soup

Ingredients

- 1/2 cup dry lentils

- Mixed vegetables (carrots, celery, onion)

- Low-sodium vegetable broth

- Herbs and spices (thyme, bay leaves)

- Spinach leaves

Preparation

1. Cook lentils and vegetables in vegetable broth.

2. Season with herbs and spices.

3. Stir in spinach until wilted.

Nutritional Information

- Calories: 180

- Protein: 15g

- Fiber: 8g

- Potassium: 300mg

- Phosphorus: 150mg

Serving Size: 1 bowl

Preparation Time: 40 minutes

6. Shrimp and Asparagus Stir-Fry

Ingredients

- 4 ounces shrimp, peeled and deveined

- Asparagus spears, cut into pieces

- Garlic and ginger, minced

- Low-sodium soy sauce

- Brown rice (1/2 cup cooked)

Preparation

1. Sauté shrimp, asparagus, garlic, and ginger.

2. Add soy sauce and stir until cooked.

3. Serve over brown rice.

Nutritional Information

- Calories: 250

- Protein: 20g

- Fiber: 4g

- Potassium: 200mg

- Phosphorus: 150mg

Serving Size: 1 serving

Preparation Time: 20 minutes

7. Eggplant and Chickpea Stew

Ingredients

- 1 cup cubed eggplant

- 1/2 cup cooked chickpeas

- Diced tomatoes

- Onion and garlic, minced

- Herbs and spices (cumin, coriander, paprika)

- Quinoa (1/2 cup cooked)

Preparation

1. Sauté eggplant, chickpeas, tomatoes, onion, and garlic.

2. Season with herbs and spices.

3. Serve over cooked quinoa.

Nutritional Information

- Calories: 280

- Protein: 12g

- Fiber: 8g

- Potassium: 300mg

- Phosphorus: 180mg

Serving Size: 1 serving

Preparation Time: 25 minutes

8. Tuna and White Bean Salad

Ingredients

- Canned tuna (in water), drained of ½ Cup

- White beans (cannellini), rinsed

- Cherry tomatoes, halved

- Red onion, thinly sliced

- Olive oil and balsamic vinegar dressing

Preparation

1. Combine tuna, white beans, tomatoes, and red onion.

2. Drizzle with olive oil and balsamic vinegar.

Nutritional Information

- Calories: 220

- Protein: 20g

- Fiber: 6g

- Potassium: 250mg

- Phosphorus: 200mg

Serving Size: 1 salad

Preparation Time: 15 minutes

9. Stuffed Bell Peppers with Ground Turkey

Ingredients

- Bell peppers, halved

- Ground turkey (lean)

- Quinoa, cooked

- Diced tomatoes

- Low-sodium taco seasoning

Preparation

1. Brown ground turkey, mix with cooked quinoa and diced tomatoes.

2. Season with taco seasoning.

3. Stuff bell peppers with the mixture and bake until peppers are tender.

Nutritional Information

- Calories: 280

- Protein: 22g

- Fiber: 6g

- Potassium: 350mg

- Phosphorus: 200mg

Serving Size: 1 serving

Preparation Time: 30 minutes

10. Vegetable and Shrimp Stir-Fry with Brown Rice

Ingredients

- 4 ounces shrimp, peeled and deveined
- Broccoli, snow peas and carrots are the examples of Mixed stir-fry vegetables we can use.
- Low-sodium teriyaki sauce
- Brown rice (1/2 cup cooked)

Preparation

1. Sauté shrimp and vegetables in a wok.
2. Add teriyaki sauce and stir until cooked.
3. Serve over brown rice.

Nutritional Information

- Calories: 260
- Protein: 18g
- Fiber: 5g
- Potassium: 300mg
- Phosphorus: 180mg

Serving Size: 1 serving

Preparation Time: 25 minutes

CHAPTER 3

Dinner Recipes

1. Baked Lemon Herb Chicken

Ingredients

- 4 ounces chicken breast

- Lemon juice, garlic, rosemary, thyme (for seasoning)

- Olive oil

- Asparagus spears

Preparation

1. Marinate chicken in lemon juice, garlic, rosemary, and thyme.

2. Bake until cooked through.

3. Roast asparagus with olive oil as a side.

Nutritional Information

- Calories: 300

- Protein: 30g

- Fiber: 4g

- Potassium: 350mg

- Phosphorus: 200mg

Serving Size: 1 serving

Preparation Time: 30 minutes

2. Vegetarian Lentil Soup

Ingredients

- 1/2 cup dry lentils

- Mixed vegetables (carrots, celery, onion)

- Low-sodium vegetable broth

- Herbs and spices (cumin, coriander, bay leaves)

- Spinach leaves

Preparation

1. Cook lentils and vegetables in vegetable broth.

2. Season with herbs and spices.

3. Stir in spinach until wilted.

Nutritional Information

- Calories: 220

- Protein: 15g

- Fiber: 8g

- Potassium: 300mg

- Phosphorus: 150mg

Serving Size: 1 bowl

Preparation Time: 40 minutes

3. Grilled Salmon with Lemon-Dill Sauce

Ingredients

- 4 ounces grilled salmon

- Lemon-dill sauce (yogurt, lemon juice, dill)

- Quinoa (1/2 cup cooked)

- Steamed broccoli

Preparation

1. Grill salmon until cooked.

2. Mix yogurt, lemon juice, and dill for the sauce.

3. Serve salmon over quinoa with steamed broccoli.

Nutritional Information

- Calories: 320

- Protein: 25g

- Fiber: 5g

- Potassium: 400mg

- Phosphorus: 220mg

Serving Size: 1 serving

Preparation Time: 25 minutes

4. Turkey and Vegetable Stir-Fry

Ingredients

- 4 ounces ground turkey (lean)

- Mixed stir-fry vegetables (broccoli, snap peas, bell peppers)

- Low-sodium soy sauce

- Brown rice (1/2 cup cooked)

Preparation

1. Brown ground turkey in a wok.

2. Add vegetables and stir-fry until cooked.

3. Drizzle with low-sodium soy sauce.

4. Serve over brown rice.

Nutritional Information

- Calories: 280

- Protein: 20g

- Fiber: 6g

- Potassium: 350mg

- Phosphorus: 180mg

Serving Size: 1 serving

Preparation Time: 30 minutes

5. Eggplant Parmesan with Whole Wheat Pasta

Ingredients

- Eggplant slices

- Whole wheat pasta (1/2 cup cooked)

- Low-sodium marinara sauce

- Mozzarella cheese

- Parmesan cheese

Preparation

1. Bake or grill eggplant slices.

2. Layer with marinara sauce and cheeses.

3. Serve over whole wheat pasta.

Nutritional Information

- Calories: 300

- Protein: 15g

- Fiber: 8g

- Potassium: 250mg

- Phosphorus: 180mg

Serving Size: 1 serving

Preparation Time: 40 minutes

6. Chicken and Vegetable Skillet with Quinoa

Ingredients

- 4 ounces chicken breast, sliced

- Zzucchini, bell peppers and cherry tomatoes are examples of mixed vegetables to use.

- Olive oil

- Herbs and spices (oregano, basil, garlic)

- Quinoa (1/2 cup cooked)

Preparation

1. Sauté chicken and vegetables in olive oil.

2. Season with herbs and spices.

3. Serve over quinoa.

Nutritional Information

- Calories: 320

- Protein: 25g

- Fiber: 6g

- Potassium: 350mg

- Phosphorus: 200mg

Serving Size: 1 serving

Preparation Time: 30 minutes

7. Shrimp and Vegetable Kebabs

Ingredients

- 4 ounces shrimp, peeled and deveined

- Bell peppers, cherry tomatoes, red onion chunks

- Olive oil

- Lemon juice

- Herbs and spices (thyme, paprika)

Preparation

1. Thread shrimp and vegetables onto skewers.

2. Mix olive oil, lemon juice, thyme, and paprika for marinade.

3. Grill until shrimp is cooked.

Nutritional Information

- Calories: 250

- Protein: 20g

- Fiber: 4g

- Potassium: 200mg

- Phosphorus: 150mg

Serving Size: 1 serving

Preparation Time: 25 minutes

8. Quinoa and Black Bean Stuffed Peppers

Ingredients

- Bell peppers, halved

- Quinoa and black bean mixture

- Diced tomatoes, onions, and spices

- Shredded cheddar cheese (optional)

Preparation

1. Cook quinoa and black beans, mix with diced tomatoes and spices.

2. Stuff bell peppers with the mixture.

3. Bake until peppers are tender.

4. Optional: Top with shredded cheddar cheese.

Nutritional Information

- Calories: 280

- Protein: 15g

- Fiber: 8g

- Potassium: 300mg

- Phosphorus: 180mg

Serving Size: 1 serving

Preparation Time: 35 minutes

9. Cauliflower and Chickpea Curry

Ingredients

- Cauliflower florets
- Chickpeas, cooked
- Coconut milk
- Curry spices (turmeric, cumin, coriander)
- Brown rice (1/2 cup cooked)

Preparation

1. Sauté cauliflower and chickpeas in coconut milk.
2. Add curry spices.
3. Serve over brown rice.

Nutritional Information

- Calories: 300
- Protein: 12g
- Fiber: 8g
- Potassium: 350mg

- Phosphorus: 200mg

Serving Size: 1 serving

Preparation Time: 30 minutes

10. Stuffed Chicken Breast with Spinach and Feta

Ingredients

- 4 ounces chicken breast, pounded thin

- Spinach leaves and crumbled feta

- Olive oil

- Herbs and spices (garlic, oregano)

- Quinoa (1/2 cup cooked)

Preparation

1. Stuff chicken with spinach and feta.

2. Seal and bake until cooked.

3. Drizzle with olive oil and sprinkle with herbs.

4. Serve over quinoa.

Nutritional Information

- Calories: 320

- Protein: 30g

- Fiber: 6g

- Potassium: 300mg

- Phosphorus: 180mg

Serving Size: 1 serving

Preparation Time: 35 minutes

CHAPTER 4

Snacks Recipes

1. Greek Yogurt and Berry Parfait

Ingredients

- 1/2 cup low-fat Greek yogurt

- Mixed berries (blueberries, strawberries)

- 1 tablespoon chopped almonds

Preparation

1. Layer Greek yogurt with mixed berries.

2. Top with chopped almonds.

Nutritional Information

- Calories: 150

- Protein: 12g

- Fiber: 3g

- Potassium: 200mg

- Phosphorus: 100mg

Serving Size: 1 parfait

Preparation Time: 5 minutes

2. Apple Slices with Almond Butter

Ingredients

- 1 medium apple, sliced

- 1 tablespoon almond butter

Preparation

1. Spread almond butter on apple slices.

Nutritional Information

- Calories: 160

- Protein: 3g

- Fiber: 5g

- Potassium: 180mg

- Phosphorus: 80mg

Serving Size: 1 serving

Preparation Time: 5 minutes

3. Cucumber and Hummus Bites

Ingredients

- Cucumber slices

- Hummus

- Cherry tomatoes

Preparation

1. Spread hummus on cucumber slices.

2. Top with cherry tomatoes.

Nutritional Information

- Calories: 80

- Protein: 3g

- Fiber: 2g

- Potassium: 150mg

- Phosphorus: 60mg

Serving Size: 1 serving

Preparation Time: 10 minutes

4. Hard-Boiled Egg and Whole Grain Crackers

Ingredients

- 1 hard-boiled egg

- Whole grain crackers

Preparation

1. Slice hard-boiled egg and serve with whole grain crackers.

Nutritional Information

- Calories: 160

- Protein: 12g

- Fiber: 3g

- Potassium: 90mg

- Phosphorus: 100mg

Serving Size: 1 serving

Preparation Time: 15 minutes

5. Cherry Tomato and Mozzarella Skewers

Ingredients

- Cherry tomatoes

- Fresh mozzarella balls

- Basil leaves

- Balsamic glaze

Preparation

1. Thread cherry tomatoes, mozzarella balls, and basil leaves onto skewers.

2. Drizzle with balsamic glaze.

Nutritional Information

- Calories: 120

- Protein: 6g

- Fiber: 2g

- Potassium: 200mg

- Phosphorus: 100mg

Serving Size: 1 serving

Preparation Time: 10 minutes

6. Carrot and Cucumber Sticks with Tzatziki

Ingredients

- Carrot and cucumber sticks

- Tzatziki sauce

Preparation

1. Dip carrot and cucumber sticks in tzatziki sauce.

Nutritional Information

- Calories: 70

- Protein: 2g

- Fiber: 3g

- Potassium: 180mg

- Phosphorus: 60mg

Serving Size: 1 serving

Preparation Time: 10 minutes

7. Nuts and Dried Fruit with Trail Mix

Ingredients

- Mixed nuts (almonds, walnuts, pistachios) of 1/4 cup

- 1/4 cup dried fruit (raisins, cranberries)

Preparation

1. Mix nuts and dried fruit together.

Nutritional Information

- Calories: 200

- Protein: 5g

- Fiber: 3g

- Potassium: 180mg

- Phosphorus: 80mg

Serving Size: 1/2 cup

Preparation Time: 5 minutes

8. Rice Cake with Avocado and Cherry Tomatoes

Ingredients

- Rice cake

- 1/4 avocado, mashed

- Cherry tomatoes, sliced

Preparation

1. Mashed Avocado should be spread on the rice cake.

2. Top with sliced cherry tomatoes.

Nutritional Information

- Calories: 120

- Protein: 2g

- Fiber: 3g

- Potassium: 200mg

- Phosphorus: 60mg

Serving Size: 1 serving

Preparation Time: 5 minutes

9. Yogurt and Granola Bowl

Ingredients

- 1/2 cup low-fat yogurt

- 2 tablespoons granola

- 1/4 cup mixed berries

Preparation

1. Mix yogurt with granola.

2. Top with mixed berries.

Nutritional Information

- Calories: 180

- Protein: 8g

- Fiber: 2g

- Potassium: 150mg

- Phosphorus: 100mg

Serving Size: 1 bowl

Preparation Time: 5 minutes

10. Pita Bread with Hummus and Sliced Bell Peppers

Ingredients

- Whole wheat pita bread

- Hummus

- Sliced bell peppers (assorted colors)

Preparation

1. Spread hummus on whole wheat pita bread.

2. Top with sliced bell peppers.

Nutritional Information

- Calories: 150

- Protein: 5g

- Fiber: 3g

- Potassium: 180mg

- Phosphorus: 70mg

Serving Size: 1 serving

Preparation Time: 10 minutes

CHAPTER 5

Smoothies Recipes

1. Berry Blast Smoothie

Ingredients

- 1/2 cup blueberries

- 1/2 cup strawberries

- 1/2 banana

- 1/2 cup low-fat yogurt

- 1/2 cup ice cubes

Preparation

1. Blend all ingredients until smooth.

Nutritional Information

- Calories: 150

- Protein: 6g

- Fiber: 4g

- Potassium: 200mg

- Phosphorus: 120mg

Serving Size: 1 smoothie

Preparation Time: 5 minutes

2. Green Power Smoothie

Ingredients

- 1 cup spinach leaves

- 1/2 cucumber, peeled and sliced

- 1/2 green apple, cored

- 1/2 cup water or coconut water

- 1/2 cup ice cubes

Preparation

1. Blend all ingredients until smooth.

Nutritional Information

- Calories: 80

- Protein: 2g

- Fiber: 3g

- Potassium: 250mg

- Phosphorus: 80mg

Serving Size: 1 smoothie

Preparation Time: 5 minutes

3. Tropical Delight Smoothie

Ingredients

- 1/2 cup pineapple chunks

- 1/2 mango, peeled and diced

- 1/2 cup low-fat Greek yogurt

- 1/2 cup coconut water

- 1/2 cup ice cubes

Preparation

1. Blend all ingredients until smooth.

Nutritional Information

- Calories: 160

- Protein: 8g

- Fiber: 2g

- Potassium: 200mg

- Phosphorus: 100mg

Serving Size: 1 smoothie

Preparation Time: 5 minutes

4. Cherry Almond Smoothie

Ingredients

- 1/2 cup cherries, pitted

- 1/2 cup unsweetened almond milk

- 1/2 banana

- 1 tablespoon almond butter

- 1/2 cup ice cubes

Preparation

1. Blend all ingredients until smooth.

Nutritional Information

- Calories: 180

- Protein: 4g

- Fiber: 3g

- Potassium: 180mg

- Phosphorus: 100mg

Serving Size: 1 smoothie

Preparation Time: 5 minutes

5. Cucumber Mint Cooler Smoothie

Ingredients

- 1/2 cucumber, peeled and sliced

- 1/4 cup fresh mint leaves

- 1/2 cup water or coconut water

- Juice of 1 lime

- 1/2 cup ice cubes

Preparation

1. Blend all ingredients until smooth.

Nutritional Information

- Calories: 30

- Protein: 1g

- Fiber: 1g

- Potassium: 150mg

- Phosphorus: 40mg

Serving Size: 1 smoothie

Preparation Time: 5 minutes

6. Banana Walnut Protein Smoothie

Ingredients

- 1/2 banana

- 1/4 cup chopped walnuts

- 1/2 cup low-fat Greek yogurt

- 1/2 cup water or almond milk

- 1/2 cup ice cubes

- 1 scoop protein powder (optional)

Preparation

1. Blend all ingredients until smooth.

Nutritional Information

- Calories: 250

- Protein: 15g

- Fiber: 3g

- Potassium: 300mg

- Phosphorus: 150mg

Serving Size: 1 smoothie

Preparation Time: 5 minutes

7. Peachy Keen Smoothie

Ingredients

- 1/2 cup sliced peaches (fresh or frozen)

- 1/2 cup low-fat vanilla yogurt

- 1/2 cup water or coconut water

- 1/2 cup ice cubes

Preparation

1. Blend all ingredients until smooth.

Nutritional Information

- Calories: 120
- Protein: 6g
- Fiber: 2g
- Potassium: 200mg
- Phosphorus: 80mg

Serving Size: 1 smoothie

Preparation Time: 5 minutes

8. Avocado Spinach Smoothie

Ingredients

- 1/2 avocado, peeled and pitted
- 1 cup spinach leaves
- 1/2 cup low-fat yogurt
- 1/2 cup water or almond milk
- 1/2 cup ice cubes

Preparation

1. Blend all ingredients until smooth.

Nutritional Information

- Calories: 180

- Protein: 5g

- Fiber: 5g

- Potassium: 350mg

- Phosphorus: 100mg

Serving Size: 1 smoothie

Preparation Time: 5 minutes

9. Strawberry Basil Delight Smoothie

Ingredients

- 1/2 cup strawberries

- 1/4 cup fresh basil leaves

- 1/2 cup low-fat Greek yogurt

- 1/2 cup water or coconut water

- 1/2 cup ice cubes

Preparation

1. Blend all ingredients until smooth.

Nutritional Information

- Calories: 70

- Protein: 4g

- Fiber: 1g

- Potassium: 180mg

- Phosphorus: 80mg

Serving Size: 1 smoothie

Preparation Time: 5 minutes

10. Mango Coconut Dream Smoothie

Ingredients

- 1/2 cup diced mango

- 1/4 cup shredded coconut

- 1/2 cup low-fat vanilla yogurt

- 1/2 cup coconut water

- 1/2 cup ice cubes

Preparation

1. Blend all ingredients until smooth.

Nutritional Information

- Calories: 160

- Protein: 6g

- Fiber: 2g

- Potassium: 200mg

- Phosphorus: 100mg

Serving Size: 1 smoothie

Preparation Time: 5 minutes

CHAPTER 6

7 Days Meal Plan

Day 1

Breakfast: Quinoa Breakfast Bowl

Lunch: Grilled Chicken and Vegetable Skewers

Dinner: Baked Lemon Herb Chicken

Day 2

Breakfast: Egg White Veggie Omelette

Lunch: Salmon and Quinoa Salad

Dinner: Vegetarian Lentil Soup

Day 3

Breakfast: Buckwheat Pancakes with Berries

Lunch: Vegetarian Stir-Fry with Tofu

Dinner: Grilled Salmon with Lemon-Dill Sauce

Day 4

Breakfast: Greek Yogurt Parfait

Lunch: Mediterranean Chicken Wrap

Dinner: Turkey and Vegetable Stir-Fry

Day 5

Breakfast: Sweet Potato Hash with Poached Eggs

Lunch: Lentil and Vegetable Soup

Dinner: Eggplant Parmesan with Whole Wheat Pasta

Day 6

Breakfast: Chia Seed Pudding with Almond Milk

Lunch: Shrimp and Asparagus Stir-Fry

Dinner: Chicken and Vegetable Skillet with Quinoa

Day 7

Breakfast: Turkey and Vegetable Breakfast Wrap

Lunch: Eggplant and Chickpea Stew

Dinner: Shrimp and Vegetable Kebabs

CHAPTER 7

Conclusion

Stage 3 Kidney Disease Diet Cookbook For Older Men And Women stands as a comprehensive resource aimed at empowering individuals navigating the challenges of Stage 3 Kidney Disease. This journey toward optimal kidney health is not merely a compilation of recipes; rather, it is a testament to the transformative power of mindful and purposeful dietary choices.

Throughout this book, we've delved into the intricate web of kidney function, the nuances of Stage 3 Kidney Disease, and the indispensable role that a well-crafted diet plays in managing and enhancing kidney health. The personalized stories shared within these pages serve as beacons of inspiration, illustrating that with commitment, education, and the right culinary choices, one can not only cope with the challenges but also thrive.

The understanding of kidney function, the impact of Stage 3 Kidney Disease, and the significance of a kidney-friendly diet has been unravelled in detail.

The collection of recipes, thoughtfully curated and designed, exemplifies the fusion of taste and nutrition. Each recipe is a testament to the belief that managing Stage 3 Kidney Disease need not be a monotonous journey but rather an exploration of culinary creativity that brings joy to the dining table. From breakfast to dinner, and even the satisfying snacks in between, these recipes are tailored to meet the unique dietary requirements associated with kidney health, while never compromising on flavor.

As we conclude this journey together, remember that the road to vibrant living with Stage 3 Kidney Disease is not a solitary one. It is a path walked hand in hand with healthcare professionals, nutritionists, and the support of loved ones. This book is a stepping stone, a guide that encourages continuous learning, adaptation, and an unwavering commitment to the well-being of your kidneys.

THANKS FOR READING

www.ingramcontent.com/pod-product-compliance
Lightning Source LLC
Chambersburg PA
CBHW082221290526
45794CB00009B/3621